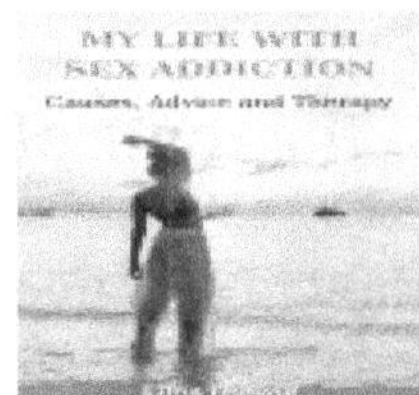

MY LIFE WITH
SEX ADDICTION
Causes, Advice and Therapy

Introduction to the topic of sex addiction

Sex addiction, also known as hypersexuality or sexuality addiction, is a controversial topic in modern psychology and psychiatry. Although the existence of sex addiction is recognized as an official diagnosis in the American Psychiatric Association's DSM-5 guidelines, the term remains controversial and is questioned by some experts. This text provides an introduction to the topic of sex addiction by highlighting various aspects such as definition, symptoms, causes and treatment options. Sex addiction can be defined as an obsessive and compulsive preoccupation with sexual thoughts, fantasies and actions. Individuals with sex addiction often have an excessive desire for sexual acts and may experience an intense craving for sexual gratification. Sex addiction can manifest itself in a variety of ways, including frequent masturbation, excessive pornography use, uncontrolled sexual relationships, or other forms of risky sexual behavior. A diagnosis of sex addiction can be difficult to make, as it is often difficult to distinguish between normal sexual behavior and unhealthy behavior. Most people have sexual fantasies or acts from time to time that are not compulsive or harmful. The difference with sex addiction is that the behavior interferes with a person's ability to go about their daily life, such as difficulties at work, in relationships, or in other areas of life. In addition to an uncontrollable desire for sexual activity, symptoms of sex addiction include a persistent preoccupation with sexual thoughts and fantasies, loss of control over one's sexual behavior, a severe impact on quality of life, and an increase in risky behaviors such as sexual activity with unfamiliar partners or unsafe sexual practices. The causes of sex addiction are not yet fully understood, but it is assumed that biological, psychological and social factors play a role. Some studies have shown that changes in the brain due to neurotransmitters such as dopamine and serotonin as well as hormonal changes can influence sexual desire and behavior. Psychological factors such as childhood trauma or stress can also play a role. Social factors such as the influence of media that portray sexuality as a constant presence may also be a factor.

Treatment options for sex addiction vary depending on individual needs. In some cases, therapy based on cognitive-behavioral therapy (CBT) can help control the behavior and develop healthy coping strategies.

What is sex addiction?

Sex addiction, also known as hypersexuality or sexual addiction, is a mental disorder characterized by an excessive, uncontrolled and compulsive urge for sexual activity. Those affected are often unable to stop engaging in sexual activity, even if this has a negative impact on their health, lives and relationships. The disorder affects men and women equally and can occur in people of all ages. There are many symptoms of sex addiction, and they can vary from person to person. Some signs to look out for are: An excessive sexual desire and behavior that is often associated with feelings of guilt, shame and anxiety. A strong focus on sexuality, even when there are other important things that need to be done. Inability to control sexual behavior, even when it has negative consequences. Frequent use of pornography or prostitution. A diminished interest in other activities that normally bring pleasure. Frequent sexual relationships, even with people they barely know. Focusing excessively on sexual experiences to cope with unpleasant feelings such as depression, anxiety or stress. Withdrawal symptoms when they have no access to sexual activity, such as irritability, restlessness, insomnia or depression. The causes of sex addiction are not yet fully understood, but it is thought that a combination of factors contribute to it. Some of the factors associated with the development of sex addiction include Genetic predisposition: It has been found that some people are more prone to sexually addictive behaviors because of their genes. Early experiences: Sexual experiences during childhood or adolescence can contribute to a person developing increased sexual desire later in life. Traumatic experiences: Traumatic experiences such as abuse or sexual assault can cause a person to develop increased sexual desire. Neurotransmitters: An imbalance in certain neurotransmitters such as dopamine and serotonin can cause a person to develop increased sexual desire. Psychological factors:

Low self-esteem, anxiety, depression or other mental illnesses can contribute to a person developing increased sexual desire. Sex addiction can have a serious impact on the lives of those affected. Relationships can suffer as those affected find it difficult to maintain intimacy and emotional connections.

The history of sex addiction

The history of sex addiction is a long and complex one, dating back to the earliest times of mankind. Sexual obsessions and behaviors were considered normal and even curative in many cultures, while in other cultures sexual behavior was strictly regulated and taboo. The modern concept of sexual addiction dates back to the 19th century, when medical doctors and psychiatrists began to study the sexual obsessions and behaviors of some of their patients. One of the earliest descriptions of sexual addiction was published in 1877 by French physician Dr. Jean-Martin Charcot, who treated a patient named "Anna O." who suffered from a variety of mental and physical disorders, including a seemingly compulsive sexuality. In the decades that followed, other doctors and psychiatrists began to look more closely at the subject. The psychoanalysis of Sigmund Freud, which emerged in the early 1900s, emphasized the role of sexuality in human life and its relationship to mental disorders such as neurosis and hysteria. Freud argued that sexual obsessions and behaviors were often based on deep-rooted psychological conflicts stemming from unresolved childhood conflicts. During the 1960s and 1970s, psychologists and psychiatrists began to view sexual dependence and addiction as separate disorders. The first scientific studies of sexual addiction were conducted in the late 1970s, when American psychiatrist Dr. Patrick Carnes conducted a study on sexual addiction that was published in his groundbreaking book "Out of the Shadows". In recent decades, the understanding of sex addiction has evolved. Today, it is considered a mental disorder characterized by a compulsive and uncontrollable sexual addiction to certain behaviors or substances. These behaviors can include a variety of sexual acts, such as: constant viewing of pornography, excessive masturbation, frequent changes of sexual partners, visiting prostitutes or constant searching for sexual contacts on the Internet. An important factor in the development of sex addiction is the presence of underlying psychological or emotional problems such as depression, anxiety or post-traumatic stress disorder. Some studies have also shown that there may be a genetic predisposition to sexual addiction. Treatment for sexual addiction can involve a combination of therapy and medication. Therapy can help treat underlying psychological or emotional problems and support those affected.

How common is sex addiction and who is affected?

Sex addiction, also known as hypersexuality or sexual addiction, is a term that refers to an excessive desire for sexual acts and activities. It is a form of obsessive-compulsive disorder and can have a serious impact on the lives of those affected. In this article, we will look at the prevalence of sex addiction and the people affected by it. It is difficult to determine the exact prevalence of sex addiction, as many people are afraid to talk about it or may not be aware that they have a problem. According to a 2021 study, an estimated 3 to 6 percent of the population has a sexual addiction. The prevalence rate is higher among men than women. Sex addiction can affect people of all ages, genders and backgrounds. However, there are certain factors that can increase the risk of developing this disorder. Some of the risk factors are: Mental illness, such as depression, anxiety or PTSD .Abuse of drugs or alcohol Previous sexual trauma Childhood problems, including abuse or neglect Relationship problems or intimate issues People who suffer from these risk factors have a higher risk of developing sexual addiction. The effects of sexual addiction can be severe and impact the lives of the person affected and their loved ones.

Relationship problems

Problems at work or school Financial difficulties due to spending on sexual activity or prostitutes Physical problems due to excessive sexual activity or risky behavior such as unprotected sex Shame, guilt and stigma It is important to note that sex addiction is a treatable disorder. There are various therapeutic approaches that can help, such as cognitive behavioral therapy, group therapy and medication. However, it is important that the person affected takes the first step and seeks help. Overall, sex addiction is a common disorder that can affect people of all ages, genders and backgrounds. There are certain risk factors that increase the risk of developing it, and the effects can be severe. Fortunately, there are several treatment options that can help sufferers improve their lives and maintain their sexual health. The effects of sex addiction on the sufferer's life Sex addiction, also referred to as hypersexuality, is a mental disorder in which a person has an excessive desire for sexual activity, resulting in recurring behaviors that can be detrimental to the normal daily activities and obligations in the sufferer's life. The effects of sex addiction on the person's life can be significant, ranging from physical and emotional impairment to social and occupational problems. Physical effects: A person suffering from sex addiction may experience physical effects such as fatigue, sleep disturbances, lack of energy and physical strength due to lack of sleep and physical exhaustion from frequent sexual activity. Frequent sexual activity can also weaken the immune system, making the person more susceptible to disease and infection. There is also a risk of sexually transmitted infections or unwanted pregnancy if no protective measures are taken during sexual behavior. Emotional effects: Sex addiction can also have a variety of emotional effects. People who suffer from sex addiction may have difficulty forming and maintaining close relationships. The frequent search for sexual gratification can cause the sufferer to become emotionally distant and have difficulty connecting with other people. Feelings of guilt, shame and anxiety can also lead to emotional problems that can affect the sufferer's self-esteem. Social impact: Sex addiction can also have social repercussions that can severely impact the sufferer's life. People who suffer from sex addiction may have difficulty forming and maintaining intimate relationships. They may also have trouble succeeding at work or school, as their addiction affects their behavior and ability to focus on tasks and be productive. People with sex addiction may also have difficulty forming healthy friendships because their addiction affects their behavior and interferes with their ability to maintain a relationship. Occupational effects: The impact of sex addiction on a person's professional life can also be significant. People who suffer from sex addiction may have difficulty doing their jobs as their addiction affects their behavior and causes them to have difficulty focusing on their work. Job loss and financial difficulties can be the consequences if the addiction is not treated.

The effects of sex addiction on the person's relationships

Sex addiction, also known as hypersexuality, is a condition in which a person has an uncontrollable desire for sexual activity. This addiction can occur in both men and women and can have a significant impact on the person's relationships. In this article, we will take a closer look at the effects of sex addiction on relationships. First of all, it is important to understand that sex addiction is a disease and that sufferers have no control over their behavior. They feel overwhelmed by their desire for sexual activity and are unable to limit or stop their behavior, even when they know it is affecting their relationships. One of the effects of sex addiction on relationships is a feeling of dissatisfaction and neglect from the partner. The person affected cannot satisfy their sexual needs without fulfilling their desire for sexual activity, which can lead to conflict in the relationship. The partner may feel that he or she is not enough or is unable to fulfill the sexual needs of the person affected. Another important factor is the guilt and shame that often accompany sex addiction. Affected individuals may feel guilty because they feel that they are betraying their relationship and their partner by engaging in sexual activity outside of their relationship. This can lead to a distancing of the partner, which further strains the relationship. The effects of sex addiction on relationships can also lead to the affected person sabotaging their partnerships. They may seek sexual activity with other people to satisfy their addiction, jeopardizing their existing relationship. This can lead to a loss of trust and a breakdown in the relationship. Another problem with sex addiction is that sufferers often try to hide their addiction. They may isolate themselves and withdraw in order to fulfill their sexual needs, which leads to a distancing from their partner. The person affected may also feel ashamed and avoid talking about their addiction, which can lead to further isolation and alienation. The effects of sex addiction on relationships can also affect the health of the partner. Sex addiction can lead to unprotected sex, which increases the risk of sexually transmitted infections. It can also lead to emotional problems, as the partner may feel that he or she is not valued or respected. However, there are steps that sufferers and partners can take to deal with the impact of sex addiction on relationships.

The impact of sex addiction on society

Sex addiction is a condition in which a person constantly or repeatedly engages in sexual behavior that interferes with their life or affects the quality of life of those around them. It is a serious mental disorder that can affect all aspects of the person's life, including their relationships, work and health. In addition, sex addiction also has an impact on society as a whole. One of the direct effects of sex addiction on society is the increase in unwanted pregnancies and sexually transmitted diseases. People who are sexually addicted tend to engage in risky behavior, such as having unprotected sex with many different partners. This increases the risk of unwanted pregnancies and diseases such as HIV, syphilis and gonorrhea. Sex addiction can also lead to relationship problems. Those affected often find it difficult to maintain intimate and trusting relationships. They can be unreliable and unfaithful, which hurts the partner and destroys trust. This can lead to the partner withdrawing from the relationship or even ending the relationship. Sex addiction can also lead to financial difficulties. Those affected often spend a lot of money on pornographic material or prostitutes. This can lead to them accumulating debts or even getting into financial difficulties. In some cases, it can even lead to them committing criminal acts to raise money. The impact of sexual addiction on society can also be emotional. People affected by sexual addiction often have feelings of shame and can isolate themselves. They have difficulty seeking support and help and often feel stigmatized and left alone. This can lead to them suffering from depression and anxiety, which can also affect their work and social life. Another factor that contributes to the impact of sex addiction on society is the portrayal of sexuality in the media. Pornography and other sexual content is often portrayed very explicitly and can be addictive. This can lead to people becoming sex addicts and engaging in risky behavior, which in turn has an impact on society. There are also effects on the world of work. People who are sexually addicted may have difficulty concentrating on their work or doing it at all. They may be late or absent frequently, leading to problems in the workplace. In some cases, it can even cause them to lose their job. The effects of sex addiction on society can also be moral.

The differences between sex addiction and hypersexuality

Sex addiction and hypersexuality are terms that are often confused or used interchangeably, but there are differences between the two conditions. Both terms describe a condition in which a person's sexual desire gets out of control and interferes with their life. It is important to understand that these conditions should not be viewed as a moral failing or character flaw, but as a medical condition that can be treated. Sex addiction is also referred to as Hypersexual Disorder and is a condition in which a person has an uncontrollable desire for sex. Sex addiction can lead to a person acting out their sexual desires, although this can have a negative impact on their relationships and life. Sex addiction is considered a compulsive disorder and is similar to other types of addiction such as alcoholism or drug addiction. Hypersexuality is a condition in which a person has an excessive sexual desire. However, it can also include other behaviors, such as excessive masturbation, excessive use of pornography, or other sexual behaviors that can interfere with the person's life. Hypersexuality can also be a symptom of other disorders such as bipolar disorder, schizophrenia or Parkinson's disease. One difference between sex addiction and hypersexuality is that sex addiction is often seen as a disorder in its own right, whereas hypersexuality tends to be seen as a symptom of another disorder. A person with hypersexuality may also have other symptoms that indicate an underlying disorder. Another difference is that sex addiction usually leads to social withdrawal and isolation, while hypersexuality often leads to impulsive behavior and risky decisions. People with sex addiction often have difficulty maintaining relationships or forming close bonds with other people. They may also withdraw socially in order to act out their sexual desires. In contrast, hypersexuality can lead to risky sexual behavior, such as unprotected sex or sex with multiple partners. It can also lead to other unhealthy behaviors, such as gambling addiction or substance abuse. Treatments for sex addiction and hypersexuality can differ. A common treatment method for sex addiction is behavioral therapy, which aims to change behavior and manage negative thoughts and emotions. Medication can also be used to treat sex addiction. For hypersexuality, treating the underlying disorder causing the symptom can be a successful method. Again, behavioral therapy can be used to reduce unhealthy sexual behavior. Medication can also be used to treat hypersexuality.

The symptoms and characteristics of sex addiction

Sex addiction, also known as hypersexuality or compulsive sexual behavior, is a disorder characterized by recurring intense sexual thoughts, fantasies or behaviors. People who suffer from sex addiction have difficulty controlling their sexuality and may experience uncontrollable sexual impulses regardless of the consequences. The symptoms and characteristics of sex addiction can vary from person to person, but in general, there are certain signs that may indicate the presence of the disorder. A common characteristic of sex addiction is the urge to constantly have sex or engage in sexual activity. This can lead to a disruption in daily life, as sufferers may neglect their work, relationships and other commitments due to their compulsive sexual behavior. They may also have difficulty controlling their thoughts and feelings and stopping their sexual behaviors, even if they feel ashamed, guilty or experience negative consequences. Another characteristic of sex addiction is the use of pornography or sexual activity as a coping mechanism for emotional problems. People with sex addiction may use sexual activity as a means of relaxation, distraction or coping with anxiety or depression. They may also engage in sexual activity to experience positive feelings such as pleasure and ecstasy. People with sex addiction often have difficulty maintaining healthy relationships. They may have difficulty forming or maintaining intimate relationships, as they often prefer sexually oriented relationships and have difficulty forming emotional attachments. They may also have problems regulating their sexuality within a relationship and tend to engage in uncontrolled sexual behaviors, even if this can lead to conflict or separation. Other characteristics of sex addiction may include: A strong desire to repeatedly have sexual activity, even if it has negative consequences An excessive desire for sexual fantasies and thoughts that are difficult to control A fixation on certain sexual activities or preferences that can interfere with other aspects of life A use of sex as a means of self-affirmation or overcoming self-doubt A neglect of work, social obligations or other important responsibilities in favor of sexual activities A risk of having unprotected sex or contracting sexually transmitted diseases A risk of being a victim of sexual abuse or harassment or being in dangerous situations.

The causes of sex addiction

Sex addiction, also known as hypersexuality or excessive sexuality, is a condition in which a person has an excessive desire for sexual activity. The causes of sex addiction are complex and can vary from person to person. In this article, we will explore some of the most common causes of sex addiction. One of the most common causes of sex addiction is early trauma. People who have experienced childhood sexual abuse or other forms of traumatization may develop an uncontrollable desire for sexual activity later in life. This can be a kind of coping mechanism to repress or overcome the trauma. Another possible cause of sex addiction is a disorder in the brain's reward system. In people with such a disorder, the desire for sexual activity can become so strong that it becomes a compulsion. This can be caused by an addiction to endorphins and dopamines, the neurotransmitters responsible for the feeling of happiness. Another factor that can contribute to the development of sex addiction is the availability of pornography.

With the increase in online pornography in recent years, it has become much easier for people to access sexually explicit content anytime, anywhere. This can lead to an addiction to pornography and an increased desire for sexual activity. Stress and anxiety can also play a role in the development of sex addiction. People who suffer from chronic stress or anxiety may use sex as a coping mechanism to relax or distract themselves. This can lead to an uncontrollable desire for sexual activity. Another possible cause of sex addiction is an impulse control disorder. People with such a disorder may have difficulty controlling their actions and act impulsively. This can lead to them developing uncontrollable sexual behaviors. Another factor that can contribute to the development of sex addiction is low self-esteem and self-worth. People who have a negative self-image may try to boost their self-esteem through sexual activity. This can lead to an uncontrollable desire for sexual activity. Another possible cause of sex addiction is an attachment disorder. People with such a disorder may have difficulty forming and maintaining close relationships. This can lead them to use sexual relationships as a substitute for emotional attachments. There is also a genetic component to the development of sex addiction.

The role of trauma and abuse in the development of sex addiction Sex

Addiction, also known as hypersexuality or excessive sexuality, is a condition in which a person has excessive sexual desire and cannot control that desire. It is a topic that is often taboo in public and not understood by many people. In many cases, sex addiction can stem from trauma and abuse in childhood or adulthood. Trauma and abuse can contribute to sex addiction in different ways. For example, traumatic events can cause a person to try to avoid pain or emotions through sexual behavior. Sexual behavior may also serve as a way to self-soothe or as a way to gain control in a situation where the person otherwise has no control. In addition, childhood abuse can lead to a confusion of sexual drive that results in sexual behaviors that can become problematic later in life. For example, victims of sexual abuse may replicate the behavior they experienced in adulthood by abusing their own sexual partners or developing unhealthy sexual practices. Another way that trauma and abuse can contribute to sex addiction is that it can affect the person's self-esteem. Low self-esteem can cause a person to view sexual behavior as a way to validate themselves and feel better about themselves. Sexual activity can also serve as a way to gain the attention and validation of others. It is important to note that not everyone who has experienced trauma or abuse will necessarily become sexually addicted. Sex addiction is a complex issue that is influenced by many factors, including biological, psychological and social factors. There are also other factors that can contribute to the development of sex addiction. For example, a person may develop excessive sexual desire due to addiction or obsessive-compulsive disorder. Also, a person going through a difficult breakup or divorce may tend to use sexual activity as a way to cope with emotional stress. Treating sex addiction can be difficult, as there is no single method that is effective for all patients. In many cases, a combination of psychotherapy, medication and support groups may be most effective. Psychotherapy can help uncover deep roots of trauma and abuse that lead to unhealthy behaviors, and can also teach techniques for coping with stress and boosting self-esteem. Medication can be used to reduce sexual desire and control the symptoms of hypersexuality.

The diagnosis of sex addiction

Sex addiction, also known as hypersexuality, is a controversial topic because the lines between healthy sexual behavior and addictive sexual behavior are blurred. There are also no clear diagnostic criteria for sex addiction, which makes it difficult to make an accurate diagnosis. Sex addiction is usually defined as a compulsive behavior in which sexual activity is so intense that it interferes with the person's life. It is important to note that sex addiction is not only characterized by excessive masturbation or sexual activity, but also by obsessive thoughts about sex, obsessions with pornography, and inappropriate sexual behavior. It is important to understand that sexual needs and desires are usually part of normal human behavior and do not necessarily indicate addiction. However, an indicator of sexual addiction is when the sexual behavior or thoughts disrupt the daily routine of life, interfere with relationships, and lead to social isolation and emotional instability. There are no standard criteria for diagnosing sex addiction, as it is not a recognized mental disorder. However, some researchers have suggested that certain criteria must be met in order to make a diagnosis of sex addiction. One way to diagnose sex addiction is to use the American Psychiatric Association (APA) criteria for impulse control disorders, as these behaviors have similarities to sexual addiction. The APA defines impulse control disorders as recurring acts that disrupt the person's life and are the result of an uncontrollable impulse. Another approach is to use the Sexual Addiction Screening Test (SAST), a questionnaire developed by researchers to identify the presence of addictive behaviors related to sexuality. The test includes 25 questions related to different areas of sexual behavior, including masturbation, pornography and sexual activity. Although there is no official diagnosis for sexual addiction, there are a growing number of therapists and professionals who specialize in the treatment of sexually addictive behaviors. These professionals can conduct a thorough assessment of the patient's behavior and provide specific therapies aimed at treating the underlying causes of the addiction and helping the patient develop healthy relationships with sexual activity. Treatments for sex addiction typically include cognitive behavioral therapy, group therapy, and medication.

The treatment of sex addiction

Psychotherapy Sex addiction, also known as hypersexuality or sexual addiction, is a condition in which people have excessive sexual desire that interferes with their lives and can lead to serious problems. Sex addiction can cause people to engage in risky sexual behavior, interfere with their relationships and professional lives, and put their health at risk. Psychotherapy is an effective treatment for sex addiction that can help people understand and overcome their problems. Treating sex addiction through psychotherapy involves different approaches that can be adapted according to the patient's individual needs. An important aspect of treatment is education about sex addiction and its effects. The therapist helps the patient understand their thoughts and behaviors that lead to sexual addiction. He also helps to identify triggers, such as stress, boredom or loneliness, which can increase sexual desire. Another important form of therapy for sex addiction is behavioral therapy. This involves identifying and changing behaviors that lead to sexual behaviors that have a negative impact on the patient's life. This can be achieved through methods such as exposure therapy, where the patient is exposed to triggers in a slow and controlled way in order to understand and control their reactions. Cognitive therapy is another approach in the treatment of sex addiction. It involves identifying irrational thoughts and beliefs that reinforce sexual desire. The therapist helps the patient to analyze their thoughts and develop alternative thoughts and beliefs that help to reduce sexual desire. Family therapy can also be useful in the treatment of sex addiction. The aim is to understand and improve relationships and dynamics within the family. Better communication and an open approach to problems can help to increase understanding and support of the family, which in turn can help to overcome sex addiction. Another form of therapy that can be used in the treatment of sex addiction is group therapy. Here, people with similar problems meet and share their experiences and strategies for overcoming the addiction. This can help to increase the understanding and compassion of group members and strengthen the patient's confidence and motivation. Treating sex addiction often requires patience and time, as behavioral and thought patterns that led to the addiction are often deeply ingrained.

The medication

Medication Sex addiction, also known as hypersexuality, is a complex and difficult issue that affects many people. It is defined as an excessive sexual desire or behavior that leads to personal or social consequences. Although treatment for sex addiction usually involves a combination of therapy, support groups and behavior modification, medication can also play an important role. In this article, we will look at different types of medication that can be used to treat sex addiction. Antidepressants Antidepressants are a group of medications used to treat depression and anxiety. Some types of antidepressants can also be used to treat sex addiction. Serotonin reuptake inhibitors (SSRIs) are a commonly prescribed class of antidepressants that can also be used for sexual disorders. These medications can help reduce sexual desire and improve impulse control. They are often prescribed in low doses and can take a few weeks to take effect. Antipsychotics Antipsychotics are medications used to treat psychotic disorders such as schizophrenia and bipolar disorder. Some types of antipsychotics can also be used to treat sex addiction. These drugs can help to reduce sexual desire and improve control over sexual impulses. They are often prescribed in higher doses than antidepressants and can take a few weeks to take effect. However, it is important to note that antipsychotics can also be associated with serious side effects, especially with prolonged use. Hormone therapy Another type of medication that can be used to treat sex addiction is hormones. Hormones such as testosterone and estrogen play an important role in regulating sexual behavior. Hormone therapy can help reduce sexual desire by lowering hormone levels in the body. However, this can be associated with a number of side effects, including decreased libido, increased bone fragility and an increased likelihood of cardiovascular disease. For this reason, hormone therapy is usually only used in severe cases of sex addiction and is closely monitored. Other medications There are other types of medications that can be used to treat sex addiction, although their effectiveness is not as well proven as the medications mentioned above. An example of this is naltrexone, a medication normally used to treat alcohol and drug addiction.

The support of sex addiction

Support groups Sex addiction is a serious condition that can have a significant impact on the lives of the sufferer and their loved ones. Self-help groups are a proven method of supporting people with sex addiction and helping them to recover. Support groups are groups of people who meet regularly to support each other and share their experiences. In sex addiction support groups, people who suffer from this disorder meet to discuss their challenges and difficulties. These groups provide a safe environment where members can open up and share their deepest fears and thoughts without fear of being judged or rejected. In support groups, members learn that they are not alone and that other people have similar problems. This realization can be a great relief and relieve the pressure that sufferers feel when struggling alone with their thoughts and feelings. It can also be very helpful to hear advice from other members who have already successfully dealt with their sex addiction. Support groups offer a variety of benefits for people with sex addiction. First, they provide a positive and supportive environment where members can express themselves freely and without fear. Second, they help members understand themselves better by sharing their experiences and emotions. Third, members learn to accept and forgive themselves, which is an important step on the road to recovery. Most sex addiction support groups are free and open to anyone suffering from this disorder. There are many different types of support groups, including those led by medical professionals and those led by former sufferers. Some support groups meet in person, while others take place online. However, support groups don't just offer benefits for people with sex addiction. They also offer many benefits for relatives of those affected. By sharing experiences and information, loved ones can learn how to help their loved one cope with their disorder. They can also learn how to protect and support themselves while helping their loved one through this difficult time. However, it is important to note that support groups are not for everyone. Some people feel uncomfortable sharing their experiences and feelings in front of others. Others prefer individual therapy or counseling to deal with their sex addiction. It is important that everyone makes their own decision about what type of support is best for them. In sex addiction support groups, there are many different approaches and techniques that can be used.

The therapy of sex addiction

Couples therapy Sex addiction, also known as hypersexuality, is a condition in which a person has an uncontrollable desire for sexual activity. This can manifest itself in a variety of ways, such as pornography consumption, frequent changes of sexual partners or excessive masturbation. People with sex addiction can suffer from a variety of negative effects, such as relationship problems, low self-esteem and depression. One way to address these issues is to consider couples therapy. In this article, we will take a closer look at the treatment of sex addiction through couples therapy. Couples therapy is a form of psychotherapy that aims to improve the relationship between partners. This can be achieved by teaching couples to communicate more effectively, resolve conflicts and meet their emotional needs. In terms of sex addiction, couples therapy can be helpful in minimizing the impact of the addiction on the relationship and helping the affected partner to overcome their addiction. An important part of couples therapy for sex addiction is working with a qualified therapist who has experience in working with sexual problems. The therapist can help the affected partner understand their addiction, identify the reasons for their behavior, and find ways to meet their needs in a healthier way. The therapist may also involve the addicted person's partner to help them understand the impact of addiction on their relationship and learn how they can best be supportive. During couples therapy, the therapist may use various techniques to help the couple improve their relationship. One of these techniques is Emotion Focused Therapy (EFT). EFT is a form of psychotherapy that aims to improve the emotional connection between partners. It can help the couple to communicate more effectively, build intimacy and create trust. In relation to sex addiction, EFT can be helpful in restoring trust between partners and supporting the affected partner to fulfill their needs in a healthier way. Another technique the therapist can use is cognitive behavioral therapy (CBT). CBT is a form of psychotherapy that aims to identify and change negative thoughts and behavior patterns. In terms of sex addiction, CBT can help identify the thoughts and behaviors that contribute to addiction and find ways to change those thoughts and behaviors.

The combination of sex addiction

Combination Therapy Sex addiction, also known as hypersexuality, is a disorder characterized by excessive sexual desire and behavior that can lead to negative effects on an individual's life. This disorder can have serious consequences, such as the development of relationship problems, social isolation and mental health issues. Therefore, treatment for sex addiction is essential. Combination therapy is often the best method of treating sex addiction. Such therapy involves the use of multiple treatment methods to achieve the best possible results. A typical combination therapy for the treatment of sex addiction usually includes psychotherapy, medication and support groups. Psychotherapy is an essential part of sex addiction treatment. It helps those affected to understand and change their thoughts and behaviors in order to develop healthy sexual behavior. One form of psychotherapy that is often used in the treatment of sex addiction is cognitive behavioral therapy. CBT can help identify and change negative thoughts and behaviors. Another form of psychotherapy used in the treatment of sex addiction is psychodynamic therapy. This type of therapy focuses on the unconscious psychological conflicts and can help those affected to understand the reasons behind their sexual behavior. Medication can also be used in the treatment of sex addiction. Antidepressants, particularly selective serotonin reuptake inhibitors (SSRIs), are a commonly prescribed type of medication for the treatment of sex addiction. These medications work by increasing serotonin levels in the brain, which can help reduce sexual desire. Support groups can also be an important part of sex addiction treatment. Support groups can provide a safe and supportive environment for sufferers to share their experiences and learn from others facing similar challenges. One well-known support group for sex addiction, for example, is Sex and Love Addicts Anonymous (SLAA). Another method of treating sex addiction is the use of relaxation techniques. These techniques can help reduce the desire for sexual behavior by helping those affected to relax and focus on other things. One relaxation technique that can be used to treat sex addiction is progressive muscle relaxation.

The difficulties of treating sex addiction

Sex addiction, also known as hypersexuality or Compulsive Sexual Behavior Disorder (CSBD), is a controversial topic in mental health research. It is a disorder in which people have uncontrolled sexual desire and often engage in sexually risky behavior. The difficulties in treating sex addiction are varied and complex. This article discusses some of the biggest challenges in treating sex addiction. Insight and acceptance One of the biggest difficulties in treating sex addiction is gaining insight and acceptance from those affected. Because sex addiction is often associated with shame, stigma and taboos, it can be difficult to seek help and admit that you have a problem. Many people with sex addiction have difficulty being honest with themselves about their own behaviors and recognizing the impact of their addiction on their lives and relationships. An important prerequisite for successful treatment is acceptance of your own problems and a willingness to accept support and help. It can help to develop a positive and open attitude towards treatment and the process of change and to free oneself from feelings of shame and guilt. Diagnosis and differential diagnosis Diagnosing sex addiction is challenging as there are no clear diagnostic criteria. There are no specific tests or examinations that can confirm a diagnosis of sex addiction. Clinical observations and the behavior of the person affected are often used to make a diagnosis. This also means that it is important to rule out other mental and neurological conditions that may cause similar symptoms, such as obsessive compulsive disorder or bipolar disorder. There is also a wide range of symptoms and behaviors that can be associated with sex addiction. It can involve a wide range of sexual activities, including masturbation, pornography, prostitution, affairs, exhibitionism or inappropriate sexual advances towards others. It may also be associated with other behaviors, such as internet or computer game addiction, alcohol or drug abuse. Multi-factor causes The causes of sex addiction are many and can vary from person to person. However, there are some common factors that can contribute to the development of sex addiction, such as childhood trauma, previous sexual experiences or brain chemistry disorders. This makes it difficult to identify and treat the exact causes of a particular individual. It is also important to recognize that sex addiction is usually not solely due to sexual factors.

The role of family members in the treatment of sex addiction

Sex addiction is a mental illness characterized by uncontrolled and compulsive behavior related to sexual activity. The disorder can have serious effects on the life of the person affected, such as problems in the relationship, professional difficulties and a disturbed self-image. The role of family members in the treatment of sex addiction is crucial. Relatives of people with sex addiction often experience an enormous burden. They often feel helpless and unsure of how to help their partner or family member. However, effective treatment of sex addiction requires that not only the person affected but also their relatives are involved in the treatment. One of the most important roles of family members is to provide emotional support to the addict. People with sex addiction can often feel isolated and lonely and may not be able to talk openly about their problems. Relatives can play an important role in encouraging the addict to talk about their problems and make them feel that they are not alone. In addition, family members can also help to get the addict into treatment. People with sex addiction can often have difficulty acknowledging their problems and seeking help. Relatives can encourage the addict to seek professional help and help them find a suitable therapist or support group. Relatives can also play an important role in coping with relapses. Relapse is a common problem in the treatment of sex addiction, and many people need support to get back on track. Relatives can help the person to pick themselves up after a relapse and show them that they still support them. It is also important that family members understand and accept the addict's needs. People with sex addiction can feel guilty or embarrassed and are often afraid to share their problems with others. Relatives can help the addict feel accepted and understood by showing them that they are not judging their behavior. Another important role of relatives is to recognize and communicate their own needs and boundaries.

Supporting a person with sex addiction can be a huge burden and it is important that family members do not neglect their own needs and boundaries. It is important that loved ones recognize their own resources and seek support from friends or family members if necessary to lessen their own burden. Finally, relatives should also make sure that they do not become co-dependent themselves.

The prevention of sex addiction

Sex addiction is a serious problem that in many cases affects the lives of those affected and their loved ones. Unlike normal sexual activity, sex addiction can negatively impact people's lives by affecting their relationships, careers and even their health. Prevention of sex addiction is therefore of great importance in order to improve people's lives and avoid negative consequences. Sex addiction is a complex and often difficult to recognize problem. It is a condition in which a person's sexual behavior gets out of control and they continue the behavior despite negative consequences. Some symptoms of sex addiction may include: constant thoughts about sex, frequent masturbation, sexual activity with multiple partners, or excessive use of pornography. A person with sex addiction may also have a desire to engage in sexual activity even if they don't really want to or if it has a negative impact on their life. To prevent sex addiction, people need to be aware of the dangers and find methods to express their sexuality in a healthy way. Here are some steps that can help:

Recognize and understand the symptoms of sex addiction

An important measure to prevent sex addiction is to recognize and understand the symptoms of the disorder. If you are aware of the symptoms, you can act faster and seek professional help before the disorder gets out of control. Reduce access to pornographic material Because access to pornographic material is so easy these days, it can be difficult to avoid sex addiction. However, it is important to reduce or eliminate access to pornographic material to avoid sex addiction. If you are having difficulty reducing access, seek professional help. Learn to deal with stress Stress can be a trigger for sex addiction, and it is important to learn methods to deal with stress. Regular exercise, breathing techniques or meditation are good ways to relieve stress and reduce the desire for sexual activity. Maintain healthy relationships Healthy relationships can help prevent sex addiction by providing emotional and physical contact. Spend time with friends and family to create a supportive environment that can help prevent unwanted sexual behavior. Seek professional help If you feel you have sex addiction or are at risk, seek professional help. Sex addiction can have serious consequences and it is important to seek help as early as possible.

The effects of pornography on sex addiction

Pornography is ubiquitous in modern society. Many people see it as harmless entertainment and a way to explore their sexual fantasies. However, there is also a growing debate about whether the overuse of pornography can lead to sex addiction. Sex addiction, also known as hypersexuality, is a mental illness in which someone engages in compulsive sexual behavior that has a negative impact on daily life. Pornography can play a role in the development and maintenance of sex addiction. This article will explore the effects of pornography on the development of sex addiction. First of all, it is important to note that not everyone who consumes pornography will develop a sex addiction. There are many factors that can play a role in the development of sex addiction, such as genetic predisposition, traumatic events in childhood or mental illness. However, pornography can be a risk factor that can contribute to a person developing a sex addiction. One of the effects of pornography on sex addiction is tolerance building. This means that a person who frequently consumes pornography will need a higher dose over time to achieve the same sexual sensations. This can lead to the person consuming more and more pornography and eventually moving on to other types of sexual behavior to achieve the same stimulation. Another effect of pornography on sex addiction is desensitization. When someone regularly consumes pornography, it can cause him or her to become more sensitive to sexual stimuli. This can lead to the person needing more and more extreme material to become sexually aroused. This in turn can lead to sexual blunting and cause the person to have difficulty maintaining normal sexual relationships. Pornography can also cause a person to become alienated from the real world. Pornography often shows unrealistic scenarios and depictions of sexuality that do not correspond to reality. If a person spends too much time consuming pornography, they may have difficulty maintaining a normal sexual relationship. It can also cause the person to have difficulty feeling empathy for other people and distinguishing between fantasy and reality. Finally, pornography can cause a person to become addicted. When a person develops a sex addiction, they may have difficulty controlling their sexual impulses. This can lead them to engage in risky sexual behaviors or engage in relationships that are harmful to them. The person may also have difficulty managing their daily life.

The impact of sexuality in advertising on sex addiction

Sexuality is omnipresent in today's society. We are surrounded by sexual images and messages in advertising everywhere. Sexuality is often used to sell products and attract the attention of potential customers. However, the frequent depiction of sexuality in advertising can also have negative effects, especially on people who suffer from sex addiction. In this article, we will look at the impact of sexuality in advertising on sex addiction, how it arises and what consequences it can have. Sex addiction is a psychological phenomenon characterized by excessive sexual behavior that has a negative impact on the lives of those affected. Sex addiction can lead to a range of problems, such as relationship problems, career difficulties and health risks. People with sex addiction have difficulty controlling their sexual behavior and often seek out new sexual experiences to satisfy their cravings. It is important to note that sex addiction is a serious psychological disorder and not simply an aversion to sexuality or a preference for frequent sex. Sexuality in advertising can increase the cravings of people with sex addiction and make them feel that they can satisfy their needs by buying products or pursuing sexual experiences. Advertising can also cause people with sex addiction to lose their inhibitions and take more risks to satisfy their sexual needs. For example, they may resort to prostitution or other illegal sexual activities to satisfy their lust. Another important aspect is that the use of sexuality in advertising can help to normalize the behavior of people with sex addiction. When sexual images and messages are constantly present in the media, people with sex addiction may feel that their behavior is acceptable and that their addiction is not taken seriously. This can lead to people with sex addiction not recognizing their problems or not seeking treatment. It is also important to note that the use of sexuality in advertising does not only have an impact on people with sex addiction. Sexualized advertising can also lead to a general culture of hypersexualization, where sexuality is everywhere and used as a means of self-affirmation and defining self-worth. This can lead to people constantly surrounding themselves with sexual messages and images, which can increase their desire and lead them to engage in sexually risky behaviors. However, it is important to note that not all people who see sexual images and messages in advertising are prone to sex addiction.

The effects of drugs and alcohol on sex addiction

The effects of drugs and alcohol on sex addiction can be severe and have serious consequences for the individuals involved and their relationships. Sex addiction, also known as hypersexuality or sexual addiction, is a mental disorder characterized by an uncontrollable desire for sexual activity. It can lead to serious problems in various areas of life, including work, social relationships and health. The use of drugs and alcohol can increase the desire for sexual activity and increase the risk of sexual misconduct. It can also lower inhibitions and cause people to act more impulsively and pay less attention to the consequences of their actions. This can lead to unprotected sex and sexually transmitted diseases. Some studies have shown that the use of drugs and alcohol can increase the risk of sexual assault. People who are under the influence of alcohol or drugs may be more likely to engage in risky sexual behaviors, including unprotected sex or sexual assault. In addition, the use of drugs and alcohol can also increase the risk of sexual dysfunction. For example, excessive use of alcohol can lead to reduced sexual arousal and impaired sexual function. Substance abuse can also lead to a decrease in sexual desire. Another potential impact of drug and alcohol use on sex addiction is the development of co-dependency. Co-dependency refers to the behavior of partners or family members who try to control or change the addict's behavior. In doing so, they may ignore their own needs and boundaries, putting their own health and well-being at risk. There are also some treatment options for sex addiction that also address the use of drugs and alcohol. Psychotherapy can help to identify the underlying emotional and psychological issues that have contributed to the development of the addiction. Medical detox may be necessary to cleanse the body of drugs or alcohol and counteract withdrawal symptoms. Inpatient rehab may be a way to overcome addiction to drugs and alcohol while treating sexual addiction. In some cases, a self-help group can also be helpful. These groups offer the opportunity to talk to other people who have had similar experiences. They can also provide an opportunity to learn new coping strategies.

The effects of certain personality types on sex addiction

Sex addiction, also known as hypersexual disorder, is a psychological disorder characterized by excessive sexual desire and behavior that leads to distress and impaired functioning. While the causes of sex addiction can be varied, studies have shown that certain personality types may be more susceptible to this disorder. In this article, we will take a closer look at the effects of personality types on sex addiction. There are different personality types that may be more susceptible to sex addiction. One of these types is the narcissistic personality type. Narcissistic people are characterized by an exaggerated sense of self-worth and have a deep need for approval and admiration from others. These traits can lead to narcissistic people engaging in excessive sexual behavior to boost their self-esteem. Studies have shown that narcissistic men are more often affected by sex addiction than women. Another personality type associated with sex addiction is the impulsive personality type. Impulsive people have difficulty controlling their impulses and tend to make risky decisions. This can lead to excessive sexual behavior as they may not be able to control their sexual impulses. Impulsive people may also be more prone to drug and alcohol abuse, which further increases the risk of sex addiction. The third personality type associated with sex addiction is the anxious personality type. Anxious people have a strong fear of rejection and criticism and tend to focus on their fears. They may also have low self-esteem, which can lead them to engage in sexual relationships to boost their self-esteem. Studies have shown that anxious people are more likely to be affected by sex addiction than other personality types. Another factor that can contribute to sex addiction is the influence of traumatic events. People who have experienced sexual abuse or other traumatic events may be more prone to sex addiction, as they may try to cope with their traumas through sexual behavior. Traumatic events can also cause people to have low self-esteem, which further increases the risk for sex addiction. It is important to note that not all people with the above personality types automatically suffer from sex addiction. There are many factors that can contribute to someone being more prone to sex addiction.

The effects of stress on sex addiction

Stress can affect the human body in many ways and often has negative effects on health. One of the possible negative effects of stress is sex addiction, a disorder that often remains hidden and untreated. Sex addiction can manifest itself in a variety of ways, including excessive pornography consumption, masturbation or unhealthy sexual relationships. In this article, we will take an in-depth look at the effects of stress on sex addiction and how to deal with this condition. Stress is often seen as a trigger for sex addiction. There is a close relationship between stress and sexuality, as sexual activity can serve as a form of stress relief. However, when a person is exposed to chronic stress, this can lead to increased sexual activity to reduce the tension. The desire for sex can become so strong that it becomes addictive and difficult to control. Stress can also cause a person to seek more and more intense sexual experiences to achieve the same satisfaction. This can lead to risky sexual behavior, including unprotected sex or sexual activity with unfamiliar partners. Such behaviors increase the risk of sexually transmitted diseases and can cause psychological and emotional problems. The effects of stress on sex addiction can also cause a person to question their sexual orientation or identity. When someone is under stress, he or she may question whether he or she is homosexual, bisexual or transgender and attempt to answer these questions through sexual activity. Such actions can lead to confusion and feelings of shame and increase the risk of further psychological problems. There is also a close relationship between stress and addiction in general. People who are under stress may be more likely to develop addictions as a way of coping. Sex addiction can be considered a type of addiction that is triggered by chronic stress. When a person becomes addicted to sex, they can often develop other addictions, including alcohol or drug abuse. Sex addiction can also lead to a deterioration in a person's relationships. When a person is addicted to sex, it can lead to unhealthy sexual relationships that can cause them to drift away from their partners. The person may also begin to neglect their work or social relationships in order to have more time for their sexual activity. If someone is suffering from sex addiction, it is important that he or she seeks help. There are many treatment options for sex addiction, including psychotherapy, group therapy and medication. Getting professional help can help minimize the effects of stress on sex addiction.

The effects of hormones on sex addiction

Hormones play an important role in regulating sexual behavior and sex drive. The hormones most associated with sexual behavior are testosterone, estrogen and progesterone. Some studies have shown that an imbalance of these hormones can lead to increased sexual behavior, also known as sex addiction. In this article, we will take a closer look at the effects of hormones on sex addiction.

Sex addiction is also known as hypersexuality and is defined as compulsive sexual behavior that interferes with daily life. The causes of sex addiction are not fully understood, but hormones may play a role. Testosterone is the most important hormone in men and affects not only libido, but also body hair, muscle mass and bone strength. Increased testosterone levels can lead to increased sexual desire. Some studies have shown that men with higher testosterone levels have an increased sexual desire and masturbate more frequently. Some men have also reported increased sexual desire while taking testosterone supplements. However, there are also studies that have found no link between testosterone and hypersexuality. Some experts believe that there are other factors that play a role in the development of sex addiction. Oestrogen and progesterone are the two most important hormones in women. Oestrogen affects libido, while progesterone has a calming effect and can reduce sexual desire. An imbalance of these hormones can lead to increased sexual desire. Some studies have shown that women with higher estrogen levels have increased sexual desire. Some women have also reported increased sexual desire while taking estrogen supplements. An imbalance of these hormones can also lead to other symptoms associated with sex addiction, such as mood swings, anxiety and depression. Women suffering from premenstrual syndrome (PMS) may experience increased sexual desire during the period of high estrogen levels. Some women have also reported having increased sexual desire during pregnancy, possibly due to changes in hormone levels. In addition to hormones, there are other factors that can lead to sex addiction. Some experts believe that a dysfunctional reward system in the brain can lead to hypersexuality. Other factors such as stress, anxiety and trauma can also contribute.

Dealing with relapse in the treatment of sex addiction

Sex addiction, also known as hypersexuality, is a serious problem that can affect the lives of sufferers. People who suffer from this disorder experience excessive involvement in sexual activity, which can have a negative impact on their relationships, work and overall quality of life. Although there are various methods to treat sex addiction, relapse prevention is an important part of any treatment. In this article, we will take a closer look at how to deal with relapse in sex addiction treatment. First, it is important to understand that relapse can be common in sex addiction treatment. Relapses can be triggered by a variety of factors, such as stress, loneliness, boredom, alcohol or drug use, relationship problems or a change in environment. It is therefore important that sufferers and their therapists prepare for possible relapses and develop strategies to prevent or manage them. One of the most important strategies for preventing relapse in the treatment of sex addiction is the identification of trigger situations. Affected individuals should learn to recognize situations or circumstances that can cause them to feel sexually overwhelmed or overly involved. These can include certain places, activities, emotions or relationships. Once sufferers have identified their trigger situations, they can develop strategies to avoid or deal with these situations effectively. Another important strategy for preventing relapse in the treatment of sex addiction is the development of coping strategies. Coping strategies can help to deal with difficult emotions such as anxiety, stress or loneliness without resorting to unhealthy sexual behaviors. These include relaxation exercises, social activities, physical exercise and mindfulness practices. Those affected should learn to integrate these strategies into their daily lives to improve their emotional stability and well-being. Another strategy for preventing relapse in the treatment of sex addiction is the involvement of family members or friends. Supportive relationships can help promote recovery and reduce the risk of relapse. Family members or friends can help reinforce positive behaviors, provide resources and offer support during difficult times. It is important that those affected build and maintain their support systems in order to be successful.

How society can help those affected by sex addiction

Sex addiction, also known as hypersexuality or sexual compulsivity disorder, is a serious condition that can severely impact the lives of those affected and their loved ones. It is a disorder in which the desire for sexual gratification is so strong that it can lead to a loss of control. The impact on the daily lives of those affected can be significant, including problems in interpersonal relationships, workplace issues and health problems. It is important that society helps those affected by sex addiction by taking both individual and societal measures. Individual measures Individual measures to support people with sex addiction include access to appropriate therapy options and psychological support programs. There are various therapeutic approaches that can help those affected, such as behavioral therapy, psychotherapy, medication and self-help groups. It is important that society ensures that the resources necessary for effective treatment are available, including financial support for people who cannot afford treatment. In addition, people with sex addiction need to be able to talk openly about their problems without being stigmatized or discriminated against. It is important that society has an open and honest dialog about sex addiction in order to raise awareness and create better support for those affected. It is important that society accepts that sex addiction is a disease and not a moral weakness or choice. Societal action Society can also help on a broader level by taking certain measures to raise awareness of sex addiction and improve the social conditions that can contribute to the development and maintenance of this disorder. One of these measures is the promotion of sex education and the elimination of myths and taboos related to sexuality. It is important that people develop a healthy understanding of sexuality in order to prevent the development of problematic sexual behaviors. Society can also help to regulate the availability of pornography. Pornography can be a trigger for sex addiction and play a role in maintaining problematic sexual behaviors. Regulating the availability of pornography can help to reduce the prevalence of sex addiction. Another social measure is to improve working conditions and reduce stress factors in the workplace.

Imprint:

Luna Ludwig
Am Anger 3
06869 Coswig

Germany
Luna-Publishing.de